contents

KT-393-792

Abdominal examination

- Ensure woman's bladder is empty
- Make sure the woman is comfortable
- Get consent

■ INSPECTION

- Examine the abdomen for the following: shape, size, scarring, rashes, striae gravidarum (stretch marks), a saucer-shaped dip at the umbilicus (suggests an occipito posterior [OP] position), bruising or trauma (? domestic violence), surgical scars.

■ PALPATION

- **Fundal** palpation – begin at the fundus (top) of the uterus with both hands to identify which pole (head or bottom) of the fetus is situated there. NB If a woman is expecting twins then two poles are likely to be felt here.

> *Tip* As a general rule, a head is harder and rounder than a bottom and is ballotable (can be rocked from side to side).

Figure 1 Fundal palpation

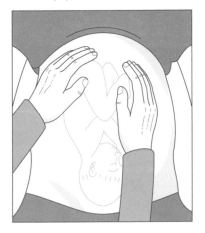

- **Lateral** palpation – with one hand support the abdomen and use it to gently push the fetus towards the other side. With the other hand (not your fingertips as this is uncomfortable) palpate from top to bottom to feel for either a firm back or limbs.

- Swap over to palpate down the other side of the uterus to confirm your findings.

Figure 2 Lateral palpation

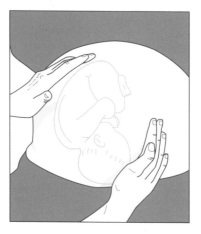

- **Pelvic** palpation
- Method 1 – using both hands as shown in Figure 3. This will enable you to confirm the fetal presentation in addition to confirming the level of engagement.
- Method 2 – the Pawlic's grip, as illustrated in Figure 4, but this is much more uncomfortable for the woman.

Figure 3 Two-handed palpation

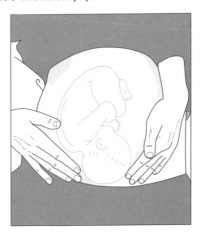

Figure 4 Pawlic's grip

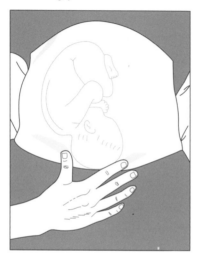

■ AUSCULTATION

- Ask about pattern of fetal movements – refer if pattern has changed.
- Current NICE guidance (*Antenatal Care* 2003, 2008a) does not recommend listening to the fetal heart at routine antenatal visits. However, it can be reassuring for parents to hear their baby.

- Using a Pinard's stethoscope count the fetal heart rate for a full minute.
- Check the maternal pulse at the same time to ensure that it is the fetal heart you are hearing.
- Following this, a Doppler device can be used.

Tip Remember not to lay the woman completely flat. The weight of the uterus can put pressure on the maternal vena cava, reducing maternal and fetal blood supply and causing supine hypotensive syndrome. As you get more practiced there is no need to have the woman semi-recumbent; she could be sitting or even standing – whichever is most comfortable for her.

Tip The fetal heart is best heard over the anterior shoulder of the fetus.

■ MEASUREMENT

- Measure symphysis–fundal height.
- Use the tape measure with the centimetres on the underside to reduce bias.
- Secure the tape measure at the fundus with one hand.
- Measure down the longitudinal axis of the uterus to the symphysis pubis.
- Plot the result on the customised growth chart.

■ EXPECTED FINDINGS

Presentation – cephalic (head), breech (bottom). (Shoulder and cord presentations are possible but unlikely to be detected by palpation alone.)

Lie – longitudinal, oblique or transverse.

Figure 5 Longitudinal lie

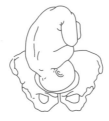

Figure 6 Oblique lie

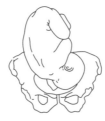

Figure 7 Transverse lie

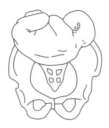

Engagement – the number of fifths of the fetal head palpated above brim of pelvis. Engagement has occurred when only two to three fifths of the fetal head can be felt.

Figure 8 Engagement

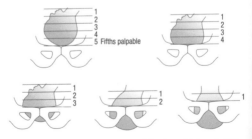

Source: Reproduced from 'ABC of labour care: Labour in special circumstances', by Geoffrey Chamberlain and Philip Steer, *BMJ* (1999) **318**: 1124–1127 © 1999 with permission from BMJ Publishing Group Ltd

Position – the direction the occiput of the fetal skull faces, e.g. right occipital anterior (ROA), left occipital arterier (LOA), left occipital posterior (LOP), right occipital posterior (ROP).

Figure 9 Fetal position

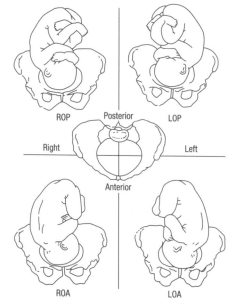

Amniotic fluid index

Figure 10 Amniotic fluid index in a normal singleton pregnancy

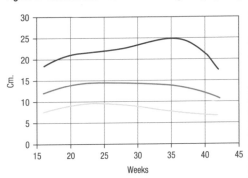

Source: This figure was published in *Atlas of Radiologic Measurement*, 7th Edition, Keats TE, Sistrom C (eds), Copyright ELsevier (Mosby, St Louis) (2001)

Measurements of the deepest pool of liquor per each quadrant of the abdomen are taken under ultrasound conditions. The total of the four measurements gives an indication of whether there is too much liquor, i.e. polyhydramnious, or too little liquor, i.e. oligohydramnios.

Anaemia

Types:
- Iron deficiency anaemia – Hb below 10.5g/dl will need further investigation

- Folate deficiency and vitamin B12 deficiency
- B12 deficiency – pernicious anaemia
- Haemolytic diseases (sickle cell, malaria)
- Anaemia following haemorrhage/infection

Need to explore the cause:
- History – diet/health/infection, symptoms
- Blood tests for those levels indicated
- Mid-stream urine (MSU)
- Faecal specimen for occult blood
- Electrophoresis

Management depends on the cause. Options include:
- Oral iron – ferrous sulphate 200mg bd/tds – can lead to intestinal upsets and black stools
- Intramuscular (I/M) – Jectofer risk of permanent staining of the skin if correct Z-injection technique is not used; allergic reactions (not often recommended)
- Intravenous (I/V) – Venofer 5ml (100mg iron) in 100ml 0.9% NaCl over 25 minutes. Need a test dose of 25mg in 25ml of solution – risk of anaphylactic shock, venous thrombosis, cardiac arrest
- 400 micrograms daily supplement of folic acid
- Alter diet to include fresh fruit and vegetables and red meat. Consider faddy eaters, vegetarians and vegans
- Drugs and alcohol can inhibit absorption
- Avoid tea and antacids if taking iron supplements as this affects absorption – need vitamin C to aid iron absorption. Haem iron is found in meat, fish, poultry – better absorption as more bioavailable
- Transfusion only if necessary – consider religious beliefs

Anatomy

■ FETAL CIRCULATION

Four temporary structures:

- Ductus venosus – oxygenated blood is directed through this structure from the umbilical vein to the inferior vena cava.
- Foramen ovale – between the atria of the heart. This enables blood flow to bypass the pulmonary circulation.
- Ductus arteriosis – lies between the pulmonary arteries and the aorta. Aids the prevention of blood flow to the pulmonary circulation.
- Two hypogastric arteries – directs deoxygenated blood from the baby's lower extremeties back through the umbilical arteries to the placenta.

Blood flow

- Oxygen diffuses across the villi of the placenta from the maternal blood.
- The umbilical vein carries the blood to the inferior vena cava in the fetal abdomen.
- The majority of the blood is diverted by the ductus venosus to the inferior vena cava. The rest passes to the liver via the portal vein.
- Deoxygenated blood travels from the liver back to the vena cava and mixes with deoxygenated blood from the lower limbs and oxygenated blood from the ductus venosus.
- Blood enters the right atrium of the heart.
- The majority passes through the foramen ovale into the left atrium and out via the aorta to the brain and body.

Figure 11 Fetal circulation

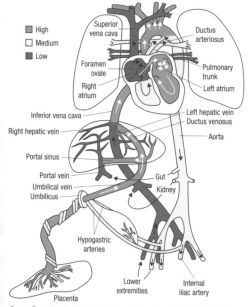

Source: Reproduced with permission from: Fernandes CJ. Physiologic transition from intrauterine to extrauterine life. In: UpToDate, Basow, DS (Ed), UpToDate, Waltham, MA 2012. Copyright © 2012 UpToDate, Inc. For more information visit www.uptodate.com

- The remaining blood passes into the right ventricle of the heart and on to the pulmonary arteries towards the lungs. The ductus arteriosus, however, regulates the amount of blood reaching the lungs by directing most of it back into the aorta.
- Blood is returned to the placenta via the hypogastric arteries, which branch off the iliac arteries.

■ FEMALE EXTERNAL GENITALIA

Figure 12 External female genitalia

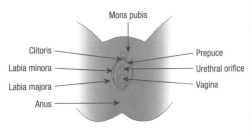

■ UTERUS

- A hollow pear-shaped organ
- Anteverted (tilted forwards) and anteflexed (curved forwards)
- 60gm pre-pregnancy to 900gm by term
- The bladder lies anteriorly and the rectum is posterior
- Three layers
  - the endometrium, which becomes the decidua in pregnancy

- ○ the myometrium: three layers of muscles (longitudinal, circular and oblique). The muscle has the unique ability to contract and retract (the fibres shorten in length) to enable birth to take place
- ○ the perimetrium.

Figure 13 The uterus

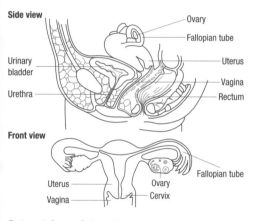

Antenatal appointments

Recommended appointments (refer to NICE 2003 and 2008a, *Antenatal Care: Routine Care for the Healthy Pregnant Woman*).

NB Women with more complex needs may require additional appointments.

APPOINTMENT	ACTIVITIES
Booking appointment before 12 weeks gestation	• Complete pregnancy records • Provide information • Blood pressure (BP) and urinalysis (including MSU) • Assess level of risk – identify any additional needs/care required • Routine booking bloods • Discuss screening options and arrange • Offer and arrange 20-week scan • Measure body mass index (BMI) • Dating scan
16 weeks	• Review and document results of screening tests • BP and urinalysis • Answer queries • Offer antenatal classes • Investigate Hb below 11g/dl – treat if required
18–20 weeks	• Anomaly scan • If low-lying placenta, arrange a further scan for 32 weeks
25 weeks nulliparous women	• BP and urinalysis • Measure and plot symphysis–fundal height

APPOINTMENT	ACTIVITIES
28 weeks	• BP and urinalysis • Bloods for full blood count (FBC) and rhesus antibodies • Investigate Hb below 10.5g/dl – treat if required • Offer anti-D prophylaxis • Measure and plot symphysis–fundal height
31 weeks nulliparous women	• Review tests from 28-week appointment • BP and urinalysis • Measure and plot symphysis–fundal height
34 weeks	• BP and urinalysis • Measure and plot symphysis–fundal height • Offer second dose of anti-D (as per trust policy) • Provide information on labour/discuss birth plan • Review any screening test results
36 weeks	• BP and urinalysis • Measure and plot symphysis–fundal height • Assess fetal position – refer for external cephalic version (ECV) if breech presentation • Discuss breastfeeding, vitamin K and newborn screening tests • Discuss post-natal care

APPOINTMENT	ACTIVITIES
38 weeks	• BP and urinalysis • Measure and plot symphysis–fundal height
40 weeks nulliparous women	• BP and urinalysis • Measure and plot symphysis–fundal height
41 weeks	• If not in labour offer membrane sweep/induction of labour • BP and urinalysis • Measure and plot symphysis–fundal height

Antenatal screening

■ BLOOD TESTS AT BOOKING

- Blood group – A, AB, O or B
- Rhesus factor – negative or positive
- Full blood count for haemoglobin level – normal range = 11–14g/dl
- VDRL (venereal disease research laboratory) – syphillis
- Rubella immunity
- Hepatitis B and HIV screening
- Sickle cell and thalassaemia

■ FOLLOW-UP BLOOD TESTS

May choose to have triple/quad test for fetal anomalies, e.g. Down's syndrome, between 10 and 20 weeks. Blood is also taken at the time a nuchal scan is performed.

Full blood count and rhesus factor are repeated at 28 weeks and 34 weeks gestation if problems arose from previous results.

■ URINE

- A mid-stream urine (MSU) test is performed at booking for asymptomatic bacteriuria.
- Tested for protein and glucose at every antenatal visit.

■ ULTRASOUND SCANS

- Booking scan up to around 12 weeks – checks viability and calculates estimated due date (EDD)
- Anomaly scan – 18–20 weeks
- If a low-lying placenta is detected at 20 weeks, repeat scan at 32 weeks gestation
- Nuchal translucency – 11–14 weeks

■ ADDITIONAL SCREENING (OPTIONAL)

- **Amniocentesis** – from 15 weeks. Amniotic fluid is extracted via the mother's abdomen and sent for DNA analysis. Identifies any chromosomal abnormalities, e.g. Edwards's, Turner's or Down's syndrome. Risk of miscarriage is 1%.
- **Chorionic villi sampling** – 11 + 2 weeks to 13 + 6 weeks. A small piece of placental tissue is extracted via the mother's abdomen and sent for DNA analysis. Risk of miscarriage is 1–2%.
- **Diabetes** – screening for risk factors only.

■ ROUTINE SURVEILLANCE

- Blood pressure at every antenatal appointment – refer if reading at or above 150/90mmHg on two or more occasions, or if marked increase from booking BP
- Dipstick urine at every antenatal appointment for protein and glucose
- Discuss pattern of fetal movements

Benefits

Benefit provision is under constant review. Current maternity benefits include:

- **Statutory maternity pay** (SMP) – paid by employers; equates to a percentage of normal wage for 39 weeks
- **Maternity allowance** – paid via benefits office for those not eligible for SMP
- **Statutory paternity pay** – two weeks' pay paid by employers
- **Healthy start** – for low-income households or pregnant women under 18. Consists of vouchers to be exchanged for healthy foods
- **Sure Start Maternity Grant** – lump sum of £500 for women on low incomes. Paid via the benefits office
- **Other benefits during pregnancy** can include free prescriptions, free eye tests (dependent on income and age), free dental treatment and widowed parents' allowance

Bishop's score for induction of labour

An assessment of the cervix used to ascertain the favourability of the cervix for induction. The higher the score, the more favourable the cervix is for a successful induction.

SCORE	0	1	2	3
Dilation (cm)	<1	1–2	2–4	>4
Length (cm)	>4	2–4	1–2	<1
Consistency	Firm	Average	Soft	–
Position	Posterior	Mid-anterior	–	–
Level	–3	–2	–1/0	+1/+2

Refer to NICE (2008b).

Blood pressure taking

ACTIVITY	RATIONALE
Wash hands	To avoid cross-infection
Ensure equipment is clean, is working and is calibrated. Also gently tap the diaphragm of the stethoscope to ensure you can hear the tapping noise	To avoid cross-infection and to ensure accurate measurements of blood pressure
Avoid taking the BP just after exertion, eating or smoking	These activities can raise blood pressure

ACTIVITY	RATIONALE
Always have the client comfortable and in the same position each time you check the BP, e.g. sitting or lying down	Posture can affect blood pressure, as can distress from being uncomfortable
Always have the extended arm well supported	If unsupported, isometric exercise (contraction of the muscles) can raise the blood pressure
Try to always use the same arm each time a recording is taken	Blood pressure can be different in each arm
Ensure the client hasn't crossed her legs and remove any tight clothing from around the arm	This can raise the blood pressure
Choose the correct cuff size (the cuff should encircle 80% of the bare upper arm)	Too small = overestimation of BP Too large = underestimation of BP
Wrap and secure the cuff around the arm 2–3cm above the antecubital fossa. The tubes should run down the centre of the inner arm. The cuff should not be too tight or too loose (see Figure 14)	To ensure accurate readings are achieved

ACTIVITY	RATIONALE
Find either the radial or the brachial pulse and inflate the cuff by closing the valve on the inflation bulb and squeezing the bulb. When the pulse disappears continue to inflate the cuff for a further 20mmHg. NB The cuff should be inflated quickly to avoid venous congestion	Avoidance of the auscultatory gap (i.e. missing some of the sounds that may affect/raise the systolic value)
Place the diaphragm of the stethoscope over the place where the brachial pulse was felt. Hold in place with one hand. The earpieces of the stethoscope should be angled forwards in the ears	Hearing may be impaired if the earpieces are angled towards the back of the ear
Slowly deflate the cuff by opening up the valve on the inflation bulb. Around 2–3mmHg of mercury per second is reasonable	To ensure there is time to hear the Korotkoff sounds. Use Korotkoff V (when the sound disappears)
Note the point when the sounds appear	To identify the systolic value
Continue to release until the sounds disappear	To identify the diastolic value

ACTIVITY	RATIONALE
Deflate the rest of the cuff quickly and remove it	To ensure the client's comfort
Avoid retaking the BP for at least 3 minutes	To avoid venous congestion
Record/plot findings and discuss the findings with the client	To aid communication and care management
Act on findings if required	To ensure appropriate management

Figure 14 Taking blood pressure

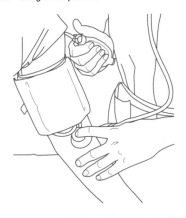

Blood values

Electrolytes

- Sodium (Na) — 134–146mmol/L
- Potassium (K) — 3.4–5.0mmol/L
- Glucose — 3.0–7.8mmol/L
  3.9–6.2mmol/L (fasting)
- Urea (age-dependent) — 4.0–8.0mmol/L
- Creatinine (age-dependent) — 0.05–0.12mmol/L
- Total protein — 63–78g/L
- Albumin — 35–45g/L
- Globulin — 25–45g/L
- Bilirubin total — 3–17µmol/L
- Alkaline phosphatase (ALP) — 35–150U/L
- Gamma GT — 5–40U/L
- Alanine transaminase (ALT) — 1–45U/L
- Aspartate transaminase (AST) — 1–36U/L
- Calcium (Ca) — 2.15–2.60mmol/L
- Total cholesterol — <200mg/dL
  <5.5mmol/L (fasting)

Blood gases

pH	7.36–7.44
pCO_2	36–44mmHg
PaO_2	85–100mmHg
Bicarbonate	22–29mmol/L
Base excess	−2 to +2mmol/L
Oxygen saturation	94–98%

Thyroid function tests

Thyroid-stimulating hormone (TSH) 1–11mU/L

Haematology

WBC	$4.5–11 \times 10^9$/L
RBC	Female $4.2–5.4 \times 10^9$/L
Hb	Female 120–160g/L
Mean cell volume (MCV)	80–100fL
Platelets	$150–400 \times 10^9$/L
Lymphocytes	25–33%

BMI

Measured at the first antenatal appointment.

Calculating BMI = weight (kg) divided by height (m)²

- Less than 18.5 = underweight
- 18.5–24.9 = healthy weight
- 25–29.9 = overweight
- 30–34.9 = obesity I
- 35–39.9 = obesity II
- 40 or greater = obesity III = morbidly obese

Booking advice

TOPIC	ADVICE
Work	<ul><li>Discuss rights and benefits</li><li>Safe to continue unless advised otherwise by a health professional or risk of occupational exposure to potential hazards</li></ul>

TOPIC	ADVICE
Supplements and diet	• Folic acid 4mg daily before conception and up to 12 weeks (5mg if high BMI or high risk of neural tube defects) • Avoid liver due to high levels of vitamin A • 10mcg vitamin D supplements if high risk, but all women need to maintain adequate stores • Avoid non-pasteurised products, e.g. soft cheese/milk • Avoid partially cooked foods, foods containing raw eggs and pâté • Drink up to 1.5 litres of non-alcoholic fluids per day • If a high BMI – don't diet and don't 'eat for two' • Aim for a balanced diet with fruit, vegetables, protein, carbohydrates, vitamins and minerals • Women who normally fast for reasons of faith should be discouraged from fasting
Prescribed medicines	• Seek medical advice as may need different medication • Avoid taking over-the-counter drugs
Recreational drugs	• Help should be sought to reduce/stop use • See section on substance misuse
Exercise	• Inform of risks associated with contact sports and scuba diving • Mild to moderate exercise is beneficial • Encourage pelvic floor exercises

TOPIC	ADVICE
Alcohol and smoking	<ul><li>Avoidance is optimal</li><li>Reduce number of cigarettes if can't stop</li><li>Limit to one unit of alcohol per day but still carries risks to the fetus</li></ul>
Travel	<ul><li>Check with airlines for maximum gestation permitted on aircraft – ensure appropriate insurance cover</li><li>Higher risk of deep vein thrombosis (DVT) on long journeys and flights – support stockings</li><li>Correct use of seatbelts – above and below bump, NOT across</li></ul>
Domestic abuse	<ul><li>Should be asked on three separate occasions of risks if able – aim to get the woman on her own on at least one occasion</li><li>Provide contact numbers of support group/safeguarding team</li></ul>
Intercourse	<ul><li>Safe in pregnancy</li></ul>
Infections	<ul><li>Avoid changing cat litter trays, gardening without gloves, handling lambs</li><li>Seek medical advice if exposed to chicken pox or rubella</li><li>Careful hand-washing to minimise spread of strep A</li></ul>
General health	<ul><li>Visit the dentist, as pregnancy can affect teeth and gums – free care in pregnancy</li></ul>

British Sign Language

Figure 15 The two-handed finger spelling alphabet

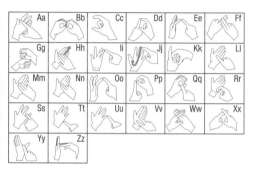

Source: From British Sign Language Resources, www.british-sign.co.uk. Used with permission

Calculating Estimated Due Dates

28-day cycle = LMP + 7 days and 9 months
32-day cycle = LMP + 4 days and 9 months
22-day cycle = LMP + 7 days and 9 months then − 4 days
Example – LMP = 1/5/2011 with a 28-day cycle
    EDD = 8/2/2012

Cholestasis

An increasingly occurring condition which develops in pregnancy and can result in stillbirths.

Characterised by intense pruritus in the absence of a skin rash; felt most intensely on the hands and soles of the feet, accompanied by abnormal liver function tests (LFTs). May also present with pale stools (subclinical steatorrhoea), dark urine and jaundice.

Management
- Liver function test: aspartarte aminotransferase (AST), alanine aminotransferase (ALT) and serum bile acid (SBA) **(normal range <14μmol/L)**
- Clotting studies
- Close observation under consultant care
- Fetal monitoring
- Cardiotocography (CTG)
- Biophysical profile
- Doppler
- Biochemical profile
- Deliver at 37–38 weeks

Medication
- Topical – calamine lotion (relieves symptoms only)
- Antihistamines (relieves symptoms only)
- Cholestyramine (Questran)
- S-adenosyl-L-methionine (SAMe)
- Dexamethasone (reduces hormonal levels)
- Ursodeoxycholic acid (UDCA/Urso)
- Vitamin K (tablet)

CMACE Top Ten recommendations

1. Pre-conception care
2. Use of professional interpreters

3. Effective communication and referrals
4. Multidisciplinary specialist care
5. Basic clinical skills and training
6. Identify and manage very sick women
7. Treat systolic hypertension
8. Prevent/recognise/treat sepsis
9. Quality critical incident review
10. Quality pathology

See CMACE (2011) for more information.

CTG interpretation

There are various ways of interpreting a cardiotocographic trace, but they all consider the same components. The following nmemonic (DrCBRAVADO) is only one way.

REMEMBER! Always check the time and date are correct on the machine/trace and that the toco paddle is set at 20mmHg, which is the normal uterine resting pressure.

DR = determine risk – consider the woman's pregnancy and medical history. Is she considered low, medium or high risk and why?

C = contractions – consider the frequency (how many in a 10-minute period?), strength (on palpation) and regularity. Is there a resting gap between them or is there coupling?

Br = baseline rate – the mean level of the fetal heart rate excluding accelerations and decelerations. Normal range 110–160bpm.

A = accelerations – increases above the baseline of 15bpm or more lasting 15 seconds or more.

Va = variability – the fluctuations from baseline should be greater than 5bpm.

D = decelerations – decreases from the baseline of 15bpm or more lasting 15 seconds or more.

- Early – uniform repetitive. Onset early in the contraction and returns to baseline. Occur in second stage due to head compression.
- Variable – vary in duration and frequency and usually have a rapid recovery to baseline. Can occur at any time, caused by cord compression.
- Late – uniform and repetitive. The peak occurs after the peak of the contraction. Caused from a delay in placental perfusion.
- Prolonged deceleration – an abrupt decrease in the heart rate lasting 60 seconds or more.

O = overall assessment and plan – is the CTG:

- **Normal** – are all the main features reassuring? Ask yourself does it need to continue?
- **Suspicious** – is there a non-reassuring feature, e.g. reduced variability?
- **Pathological** – is more than one feature non-reassuring?

The management of these women is dependent on the overall picture and severity of any non-reassuring features.

Possible options include any or all of the following:
- Alter maternal position – left lateral is often very effective
- Check maternal observations. A sudden drop in BP (e.g. after an epidural top-up) can induce a prolonged deceleration
- Refer to obstetric team and inform shift coordinator

- Fetal blood sampling (FBS). **NB** a drop in fetal blood pH and increase in base excess is significant. FBS may be performed more than once
- Delivery

Customised growth charts

Figure 16 Example of a customised growth chart

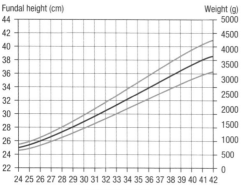

Source: Copyright Gestation Network. Used with permission

Measurements of fundal height and measurements taken at ultrasound scans should be plotted on a customised growth chart such as the one shown in Figure 16. Regular measurements will demonstrate the pattern of fetal growth. Deviations from the expected centiles require further investigation.

Diabetes

■ TYPE 1 DIABETIC WOMEN

Preconception:

- All women of childbearing age should be asked about their plans for pregnancy and referred to a specialist diabetes team for optimisation of control
- HbA_{1c} should be measured within the six months prior to conception and ideally be below 6.1%
- Folic acid 5mg supplements commenced prior to conception and for at least the first trimester of pregnancy

Pregnancy:

- Early referral to a multidisciplinary team is optimal. Team to include consultant obstetrician, consultant diabetologist, midwife/midwife diabetes specialist, diabetes nurse specialist and dietician

Booking bloods plus:

- Blood sugar and HbA_{1c}
- Urea and electrolytes
- Serum creatinine and albumin
- Thyroid function test
- Urine albumin/creatinine ratio (ACR)

Screening:

- Ultrasound scans for viability, dating scan, 20-week anomaly scan plus detailed cardiac scan/fetal echo
- Followed by serial growth scans from 24 weeks
- Full retinal assessment during each trimester using digital photography through dilated pupils. Referral to an ophthalmologist if any problems detected

- May need to do a 24h urine collection for specific amount of protein
- Monitor blood pressure
- Oedema
- Refer to the renal team
- May consider aspirin therapy or Clexane
- Agree glycaemia targets and explain importance
- Review diary at each visit and adjust insulin as required
- Prescribe glucagon and ketostix
- Give contact numbers
- Routine antenatal care to monitor overall maternal and fetal well-being

■ GESTATIONAL DIABETIC WOMEN

Develops during pregnancy only but there may be an underlying type 1 or 2. May be detected through a random blood glucose >7.2, 3+ glucose at any time or 2+ x 2 in routine urine testing, raised HbA_{1c} identified from maternal haemoglobinopathy screening or a history of polycystic ovary syndrome.

- Glucose tolerance test (GTT) arranged at booking and if normal repeated at around 26 weeks
- Dependent on the gestation, clinical picture and the results of blood sugar monitoring, may need to start on insulin or be diet-controlled
- Weekly CTGs from 36 weeks, earlier if a problem identified
- Plan for induction of labour or elective Caesarean section from 38 weeks

- If anticipating premature/early birth with the need for betamethasone/steroids, then will require sliding-scale insulin

Drug administration

■ DRUGS AND MIDWIVES/STUDENT MIDWIVES

- Appropriate training must be undertaken to administer any drug
- Qualified midwives can administer on their own initiative drugs on the Midwifery Exemptions list – see the NMC (2011) circular and Trust lists
- If trained and signed up for, qualified midwives can administer appropriate Patient Group Directives (PGDs) without prescription
- Student midwives (regardless of any prior qualifications) can administer drugs on the exemptions list **only** and only under *direct* supervision from a qualified midwife. This excludes drugs on the PGD list and controlled drugs including pethidine which need prescribing
- Drugs that were originally an exemption but moved to the list of PGDs *cannot* be administered by a student midwife
- Any drug not listed as an exemption or PGD must be prescribed by a medical practitioner
- Administration of drugs **must** adhere to the local Trust policy

■ SAFE ADMINISTRATION

Remember to check the woman isn't allergic to the drugs prescribed!

The five rights

FIVE RIGHTS	WHAT TO CHECK
Right patient	Check wristband against drug chart Confirm woman's name, date of birth and unit number
Right medicine	Check the packaging and date of expiry
Right dose	Check dose of drug on packaging against prescription chart and calculate required amount, e.g. number of tablets
Right time	Check when previous dose administered and check prescription chart
Right route	Check prescribed route is correct for the drug to be administered Check the woman is physically able to take the medication

Always check the effect of the medication following administration, e.g. has the pain relief worked, have there been any side effects?

■ DRUG ABBREVIATIONS

BD – bis die, twice daily
g – gram
IM – intramuscular
IV – intravenous
Mané – morning
mcg – microgram

mg – milligram
ml – millilitre
Nocté – night
OD – omni die, once daily
PO – per oral
PR – by rectum
PRN – pro re nata, when required
QDS – quater die sumendum, four times daily
SC – subcutaneous
SL – sublingual
Stat – immediately
Supp – suppository
TDS – ter die sumendum, three times daily

■ FORMULAS

Tablets/solutions

$$\text{Amount required} = \frac{\text{strength required}}{\text{strength in stock}} \times \frac{\text{volume}}{1}$$

Intravenous Infusions

$$\text{Rate (drops per minute)} = \frac{\text{volume to be infused}}{\text{time in hours}} \times \frac{\text{drop rate}}{60 \text{ minutes}}$$

The drop rate is found on the giving set.

$$\text{Rate (mL/h)} = \frac{\text{volume (ml)}}{\text{time (hours)}}$$

Emergencies

■ ADULT LIFE SUPPORT FOR A PREGNANT WOMAN

Figure 17 Adult life support for the pregnant woman

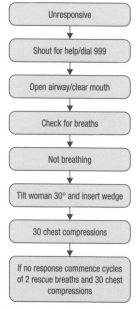

Source: Based on information from Resuscitation Council (UK) (2010) Resuscitation Guidelines, http://www.resus.org.uk/pages.guide.htm

■ ANTEPARTUM HAEMORRHAGE

Any amount of bleeding in pregnancy should be referred to the hospital.

Figure 18 Management of an antepartum haemorrhage

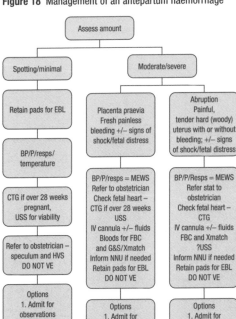

■ PRE-ECLAMPSIA

The second highest cause of maternal mortality in the UK (CMACE 2011). Can occur at any point from 20 weeks gestation. It may also suddenly develop in the postnatal period when the highest risk is within the first 72 hours post-birth.

Signs and symptoms

- BP of 150/90mmHg or more in a normatensive woman. Rule out anxiety/underlying hypertension
- + or more protein in the urine (rule out contamination and UTI)
- Oedema – more than just ankles
- Headaches – commonly frontal and not relieved by painkillers
- Epigastric pain – pain on upper right side of abdomen
- Visual disturbances – blurred vision, flashing lights
- Hyperreflexia
- Agitation/confusion, reduced urine output (oligurea) – may be eclamptic

Management

Depends on severity of symptoms.
- Mild to moderate – refer to day assessment unit (DAU) or delivery suite, recheck BP, urine (dipstick and MSU), bloods (FBC, U&Es, LFTs, clotting, ?group and save), CTG, ?Doppler scan
- Moderate to severe – as above plus strict fluid balance, 24-hour urine collection, consider delivery
- If premature may need IM steroids (CMACE 2011)

■ ECLAMPSIA

Figure 19 Management of eclampsia

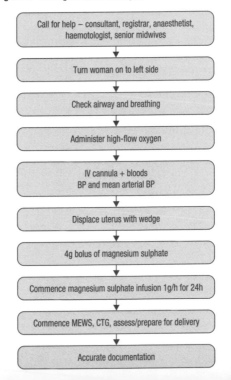

Female circumcision

There are four types:

- Type 1 – clitoridectomy: partial or total removal of the clitoris and possibly the prepuce.
- Type 2 – excision: partial or total removal of the clitoris and the labia minora, with or without excision of the labia majora.

Figure 20 Degrees of female genital mutilation

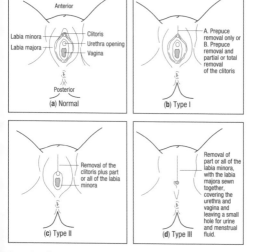

(a) Normal

(b) Type I

(c) Type II

(d) Type III

Source: http://commons.wikimedia.org/wiki/File:FGC_Types.jpg, Kaylina

- Type 3 – infibulation: narrowing of the vaginal opening through the creation of a covering seal. The seal is formed by cutting and repositioning the inner, and sometimes outer, labia, with or without removal of the clitoris.
- Type 4 – other: all other harmful procedures to the female genitalia for non-medical purposes, e.g. pricking, piercing, incising, scraping and cauterising the genital area.

Women with type 3 will need referral to a specialist midwife for follow-up care and for deinfibullation if they wish to have a vaginal birth.

Functions of the placenta

- Respiration – absorbs oxygen and excretes carbon dioxide
- Nutrition – glucose is stored as glycogen. Placental enzymes break down nutrients supplied by the mother
- Excretion – fetal waste products are transferred back to the mother via the placenta
- Protection – limited but prevents the passage of bacteria and enables maternal antibodies to pass to the fetus
- Hormone production – (a) hCG to maintain the corpus luteum until the placenta is fully formed by about 12 weeks; (b) progesterone and oestrogen; (c) human placental lactogen for glucose metabolism

Methods of induction

- *Membrane sweep* performed by midwife or obstetrician between 40 and 42 weeks gestation
- *Artificial prostaglandin* – pessary or gel – inserted into the posterior fornix of the cervix. Can take more than one dose to soften the cervix
- *Artificial rupture of membranes* (ARM) using an amnihook. Requires the cervix to be effaced and dilated enough, and the presenting part to be engaged in the pelvis
- *Oxytocin intravenous infusion* – commenced only after the rupture of membranes. Can induce contractions very quickly so sufficient analgesia needs to be considered

Figure 21 Use of an amnihook

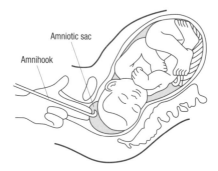

Amniotic sac

Amnihook

Minor disorders

DISORDER	SUGGESTED MANAGEMENT/ADVICE
Nausea and vomiting	• Reassure – in the majority of cases this subsides by 16 weeks • Small regular meals • Avoid fatty foods • Maintain fluid intake • Seek medical help if severe/doesn't subside • Ginger/acupressure/antihistamines may help
Varicose veins	• Elevate legs when able • Regular gentle exercise – ankle exercises if sitting for long periods • Support stockings • Avoid excessive weight gain • Report any pain or inflamed areas • Avoid tight waistbands, belts etc.
Constipation	• Increase fluid intake • Eat fibre, especially from fruit and vegetables • Avoid straining • Seek medical help if persistent as may need a mild laxative • NB can be exacerbated by iron supplements

DISORDER	SUGGESTED MANAGEMENT/ADVICE
Itching	• Keep as cool as possible • Wear loose cotton clothing • Avoid scratching • Use calamine lotion if a rash is present or skin inflamed • Seek medical help immediately if excessive, especially if located primarily on hands and feet • Prescribed antihistamines may help
Haemorrhoids	• As with constipation • Topical creams may help
Bleeding gums/ gingivitis	• Careful regular brushing of teeth with a soft bristle brush • Visit dentist regularly – free during pregnancy
Heartburn	• Small regular meals • Avoid high-fat meals or spicy foods if applicable • Milk may help some women • Sleep propped up on pillows • Antacids suitable in pregnancy can be used • Avoid coffee, alcohol, smoking and chocolate – can increase heartburn

DISORDER	SUGGESTED MANAGEMENT/ADVICE
Vaginal discharge/ thrush	• Increased discharge is normal unless accompanied by itching, offensive smell or soreness • Topical imidazole can be used to treat *Candida* infections • Cotton underwear • Maintain good levels of hygiene • Ensure partner is treated if appropriate • Avoid wearing tight trousers, jeans and tights • Wipe front to back following use of toilet

Substance misuse

Most of the following are associated with polysubstance use (using more than one at any one time); an increase in domestic violence and sexual abuse; poor attendance for antenatal care; late booking, and an increase in psychiatric disorders.

SUBSTANCE	APPEARANCE	SIDE EFFECTS	PREGNANCY ADVICE
Benzopiperazine (BZP)	Powder or tablets – oral, snorted or smoked	Affect lasts 6–8h, stomach pains, vomiting, fever, diarrhoea, fits, heart attacks Pregnancy – potential impact from risky behaviour	Illegal and unsafe; avoid during pregnancy
Caffiene	Found in coffee, tea and energy drinks	Shakes, high blood pressure, anxiety, headaches, nausea, insomnia Pregnancy – linked to miscarriage and low-birth-weight (LBW) babies	An excess is thought to be harmful for fetal growth and may cause withdrawal following the birth. Limit daily intake to no more than two cups of coffee. Legal

SUBSTANCE	APPEARANCE	SIDE EFFECTS	PREGNANCY ADVICE
Cannabis	Rolled with tobacco as spliffs, or in hash cakes	Paranoia, hunger, anxiety, panic attacks, long-term use linked to cancer and schizophrenia. Pregnancy – financial and relationship issues, premature birth, withdrawal issues for baby, sudden infant death syndrome (SIDS)	Illegal class B drug. Stop or reduce use. Refer to specialist help. Needs regular monitoring of fetal well-being and growth
Cocaine	White powder, inhaled, injected or swallowed	Highly addictive, depression, twitches, hallucinations, insomnia, violent behaviour, raised temperature and blood pressure. Can kill. Pregnancy – STDs more common, miscarriage, low-birth-weight infants, premature birth, intrauterine growth restriction (IUGR), placental abruption	Avoid where possible. Seek medical help – refer to substance misuse midwife. Use clean needles – avoid sharing equipment. Illegal class A drug. Needs sexually transmitted disease (STD) screening. May need to avoid

SUBSTANCE	APPEARANCE	SIDE EFFECTS	PREGNANCY ADVICE
Crystal meth	Small ice crystals – smoked or injected	Rapid heart rate and BP, seizures, convulsions, hallucinations, nausea, loss of appetite, tooth decay, heart attack, stroke, epilepsy, organ damage. Pregnancy – miscarriage, placental abruption, low-birth-weight babies, ? heart defects, withdrawal symptoms for baby	Illegal class A drug. Avoid during pregnancy but do not stop using suddenly. Needs a controlled withdrawal programme
Ecstasy	Coloured tablets or capsules with motifs	Effect lasts about 4–5h. Dilated pupils, confusion, paranoia, kidney and liver damage, heart disease, depression Pregnancy – ? linked to limb defects	Illegal class A drug. Avoid in pregnancy

SUBSTANCE	APPEARANCE	SIDE EFFECTS	PREGNANCY ADVICE
GHB	Clear undetectable fluid	A central nervous system depressant, therefore sedates. Risk of burns to throat and stomach. Used for date rape. Pregnancy – no evidence yet produced	Illegal. Very addictive and dangerous if taken with alcohol. Overdosing can induce coma. Avoid in pregnancy.
Heroin	Brown/white powder – injected, inhaled or snorted	Never 100% pure. Nasal damage, collapsed damaged veins, breathing difficulties, chronic constipation, stomach cramps. Pregnancy – amenorrhoea, poor nutrition, IUGR, premature birth, bleeding, fetal distress. Causes withdrawal symptoms in the baby	Refer to substance misuse midwife/obstetrician – avoid sharing needles due to risk of hepatitis B and C or HIV/AIDS. Need a controlled withdrawal programme: do not stop using suddenly Limits choices for analgesia in labour Safer alternatives, e.g. methadone

SUBSTANCE	APPEARANCE	SIDE EFFECTS	PREGNANCY ADVICE
LSD/acid	Licked off squares of blotting paper, capsules or liquid. Odourless and tasteless	Extreme fear, panic attacks, depression, speech problems, coma Pregnancy – evidence of link to low-birth-weight babies, birth defects, brain damage	Illegal class A drug. Avoid in pregnancy
Magic mushrooms	Brown-capped mushrooms	Hallucinations, nausea and vomiting, stomach pains, diarrhoea. Easily mistaken for other field mushrooms and can be fatal	Illegal class A drug. Avoid in pregnancy

SUBSTANCE	APPEARANCE	SIDE EFFECTS	PREGNANCY ADVICE
Nicotine/ smoking	One of 4000 chemicals in cigarettes/ snuff	Respiratory problems, increased heart rate, cancer, stroke Pregnancy – IUGR, premature birth, stillbirth, SIDS, often associated with consumption of other harmful substances. Passive smoking equally harmful	Reduce or stop consumption Refer to smoking cessation midwife A CO (carbon monoxide) breath test may be performed
Solvents	e.g. spray paint, glues, correction fluid – inhaled	Can be fatal, organ damage, loss of smell and hearing, nose bleeds, rashes, headaches Pregnancy – ? miscarriage, congenital abnormalities, premature birth	Not illegal but should be avoided completely in pregnancy
Speed/ amphetamines	White powder – snorted, swallowed, dissolved, injected	Very addictive, paranoia, anxiety, psychosis. If injected, risk of ulcers and gangrene	Illegal. Avoid in pregnancy

SUBSTANCE	APPEARANCE	SIDE EFFECTS	PREGNANCY ADVICE
Alcohol	Various	Accidents, cancer, liver damage. Pregnancy – fetal alcohol syndrome, premature birth, fetal abnormalities	NICE (2008a) Antenatal guidance no more than one standard unit per week. Avoid completely during first three months at least. No consumption of alcohol is optimal. When breastfeeding, one or two units once or twice a week is considered safe. Women should be discouraged from drinking and then sleeping with the baby in the bed with them

Support groups

ARC Antenatal Results and Choices 0207 6310285

Citizen's Advice Bureau 0207 8332181

Contact a Family for parents with/expecting disabled children 0808 8083555

Drinkline 0800 9178282

FSA Financial Services Authority 0845 606 1234

La Leche league breastfeeding advice and support 0845 1202918

Miscarriage Association 01924 200799

National Domestic Violence helpline 0808 20000247

NCT National Childbirth Trust 0300 3300772

NHS Direct 0845 4647

NHS Pregnancy Smoking Helpline 0800 1699169

TAMBA Twins and Multiple Births Association 01483 304442

Women at risk (FGM) 0207 2019982

Working Families (Rights and benefits) 0800 0130313

Useful websites

---

www.NMC-uk.org
Nursing and Midwifery Council

www.nice.org.uk
National Institute of Health and Clinical Excellence

www.rcog.org.uk
Royal College of Obstetricians and Gynaecologists

www.rcm.org.uk
Royal College of Midwives

www.pi.nhs.uk
Perinatal Institute

Venepuncture

Ensuring the physical and psychological comfort of the client:

- Explain procedure and obtain consent
- Use of anaesthetising creams if appropriate
- Positioning of client – seated or lying
- Privacy
- Support limb – use a pillow or armrest
- Good light source

Anatomy and physiology:

- Blood must only be taken from a vein.
- Veins of choice = basilic, cephalic and the median cubital – the superficial veins of the upper limb (Figure 22).
- Additional blood volume and a rise in body temperature in pregnancy usually makes venepuncture easier.
- Care must be taken to avoid nerves and arteries, which lie between the veins.
- The procedure must be stopped if an artery or nerve is hit.

Figure 22 Veins of the forearm

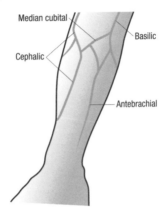

Aseptic (clean) technique:
- Hands should be washed and dried thoroughly.
- Gloves are recommended for protection and to further reduce risk of contamination.
- If alcohol swabs are used, the skin should be rubbed firmly with the swab and left to dry for 30 seconds.
- The vein SHOULD NOT then be palpated again as this will contaminate the area.
- Equipment should be disposable and needles must be sterile.
- Blood spillages must be cleaned up immediately, following local guidelines for spillages.

Choosing a site:

- The area must be free from inflammation, bruising or infection. Avoid reusing a site.
- The vessel must be easily palpated and/or visible.
- If an IVI is *in situ* the opposite limb should be used to avoid dilution of the sample.
- Ask the client if they have had any problems before – if in doubt get someone with more experience.

Equipment needed

- Receiver
- Tourniquet
- Blood bottles
- A green Vacutainer needle and plastic connector (see Figures 23 and 24); or a 21G (green) needle and appropriate size syringe
- Alcohol swab
- Gloves

Figure 23 Vacutainer® connectors

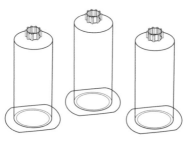

Figure 24 Vacutainer® needle

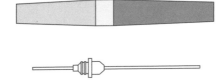

- Gauze or cottonwool and tape or plaster (note any allergies)
- Specimen request forms
- Sharps box

Health and safety:
- Aseptic/clean technique should be used at all times to minimise the risk of contamination and localised infection.
- All used equipment, needles etc. must be disposed of immediately in the nearest sharps box.
- Sharps boxes should not be overfilled, to avoid sharps injuries.
- NEVER resheath used needles.
- Treat all blood as if it is infectious.
- Report any injuries straight away and deal with them appropriately.
- Clean up any spillages immediately.

Potential problems:
- Client may feel faint or actually faint
- Needle phobias

- Needlestick injuries
- Failure to obtain blood
- Bruising
- Arterial puncture
- Nerve damage

■ PROCEDURE FOR TAKING BLOOD

- Decide on the tests to be performed
- Inform the client and obtain their consent
- Collect and assemble equipment
- Position the client comfortably and support the limb
- Wash hands and put on gloves
- Apply the tourniquet carefully, avoiding pinching the skin
- Select a vein
- Wipe the skin with an alcohol swab (if used) and allow skin to dry
- Anchor the vein with the thumb of the non-dominant hand
- Insert needle into the vein until the lumen is no longer visible
- Support needle with the non-dominant hand
- Draw back on syringe plunger or insert vacutainer bottles Swap each vacutainer bottle as they are filled, taking care not to move the needle when inserting them
- Release the tourniquet and withdraw needle
- Apply pressure immediately to site for at least 1 min. Do not bend the arm as this will cause bruising
- Dispose of waste and sharps safely
- Inspect puncture site and apply dressing
- Remove gloves and wash hands
- Label bottles and complete forms – send specimens to the laboratory

- Document which blood tests have been performed in the client's notes
- Inform the client about how she will receive the results

Vulnerable groups of women

Some groups of women will need their care specifically adapted to meet their additional needs and maintain their well-being alongside that of the fetus and baby.

Look out for:
- Sufferers of domestic violence
- Substance misusers
- Teenagers
- Older mothers
- Obese women
- Asylum seekers/refugees
- Women who don't have English as their first language
- Women with some form of disability

General abbreviations

Tip Many abbreviations are used in midwifery – however, officially only those accepted by your individual Trust should be used.

ACR	albumin/creatinine ratio
ALP	alkaline phosphatise
ALT	alanine transaminase
AST	aspartate transaminase

APH	antepartum haemorrhage
ARM	artificial rupture of membranes
BD	twice daily
BMI	body mass index
BP	blood pressure
BPM	beats per minute
Br	baseline rate
Ca	calcium
C/O	care of or complaining of
CAF	Common Assessment Framework
CRL	crown–rump length
CTG	cardiotocograph
DV	domestic violence
DVT	deep vein thrombosis
EDD	estimated due date/estimated date of delivery
EBL	estimated blood loss
FBC	fluid balance chart
FBC	full blood count
FBS	fetal blood sampling
FD	forceps delivery
FH	fundal height
FHHR	fetal heart heard and regular/reactive
FL	femur length
FM	fetal movements
G	gravida (the number of pregnancies)
H/O	history of
Hb	haemoglobin
HC	head circumference
HELLP	haemolysis, elevated liver enzymes and low platelets
HVS	high vaginal swab

IUCD	intrauterine contraceptive device
IUD	intrauterine death
IUGR	intrauterine growth restriction
IVI	intravenous infusion
LBW	low birth weight
LFT	liver function tests
LOA	left occipito anterior
LOP	left occipito posterior
LSCS	lower-segment Caesarean section
MC&S	microscopy and sensitivity
MEW/MEOW	Modified Early (Obstetric) Warning Score
MLC	midwifery-led care
MSU	mid-stream urine
NBM	nil by mouth
NVB	normal vaginal birth
OA	occipito anterior
OP	occipito posterior
P	parity (the number of births over 24 weeks)
PGD	Patient Group Directive
PO	per oral
PR	per rectum
PV	per vagina
ROA	right occipito anterior
ROP	right occipito posterior
SAMe	S-adenosyl-L-methionine
SB	stillbirth
SBA	serum bile acid
SGA	small for gestational age
SMP	statutory maternity pay
SROM	spontaneous rupture of membranes
STD	sexually transmitted disease

TDS	three times daily
TPR	temperature, pulse and respirations
U&E	urea and electrolytes
UDCA	ursodeoxycholic acid
USS	ultrasound scan
UTI	urinary tract infection
VBAC	vaginal birth after Caesarean
VDRL	Venereal Disease Research Laboratory
VE	vaginal examination
Xmatch	cross-match

References

CMACE (2011) *Saving Mothers' Lives. Reviewing Maternal Deaths to make Motherhood Safer: 2006–2008*. London: BJOG and Wiley-Blackwell.

NICE (2003) *Antenatal Care: Routine Care for the Healthy Pregnant Woman*. Guideline 6. London: NICE.

NICE (2008a) *Antenatal Care: Routine Care for the Healthy Pregnant Woman*. Guideline 62. London: NICE.

NICE (2008b) *Induction of Labour Guideline*. London: NICE.

NMC (2011) *Changes to Midwives' Exemptions*. Circular 7. London: NMC.

Shift roster

DAY	DATE	SHIFT
MONDAY		
TUESDAY		
WEDNESDAY		
THURSDAY		
FRIDAY		
SATURDAY		
SUNDAY		